EAT SO WHAT!

THE POWER OF VEGETARIANISM

VOLUME 2

Nutrition Guide for Weight Loss, Disease Free, Drug Free, Healthy Long Life

(Mini Edition)

LA FONCEUR

CONTENTS

PREFACE

Being a Research Scientist and Registered Pharmacist, I have worked closely with drugs. Based on my experience, I would suggest not to depend on drugs but to eat healthy vegetarian foods that have the power to protect you from many diseases. Vegetarian diet can add valuable and healthy years to your life. In this book, I am throwing light on the fact that how plant-based healthy vegetarian foods are the remedy to most of our daily health problems.

In *Eat So What! The Power of Vegetarianism Volume 2*, you are going to understand your food scientifically and realistically. Do not be misled by any random diet. Learn why each nutrient is important, how you can get maximum health benefits from nutrients. Learn how to prevent vitamin B12 deficiency while you are vegetarian.

You will also discover some tasty and healthy recipes to boost your health as well as satisfy your urge to eat out. Discover some simple yet recipes that anyone can cook at home. You no longer need to compromise on taste to eat healthy foods.

La Fonceur

CHAPTER 1

WHAT ARE NUTRIENTS? WHY ARE THEY SO IMPORTANT?

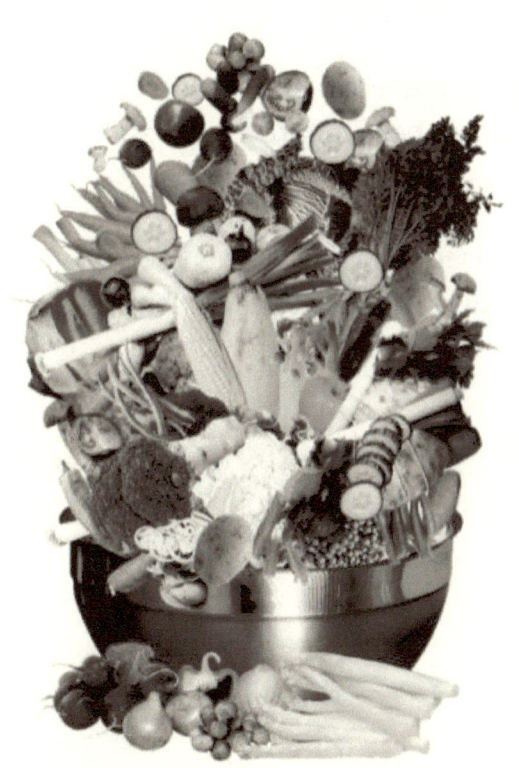

N utrients are this, nutrients are that, falla food is more nutritious, falla food should not be eaten as it is not nutritious, blah blah blah... you may have heard these things thousands of times. So many fuss about nutrition value, but the question is, what factors decide which food is more nutritious and which one is not? What makes food nutritious? The Answer is, the number of nutrients present in a food decides its nutrition value. Now, what are Nutrients?

This chapter will answer all of your questions about nutrients.

What are Nutrients?

Nutrients are:

- Substances present in our food and are essential for our life.
- Providing us energy, essential for repair and growth.
- Regulating chemical processes, and necessary for the maintenance of overall health.

I have summarised all about nutrients in the figure. We will understand each one in detail one by one in this chapter.

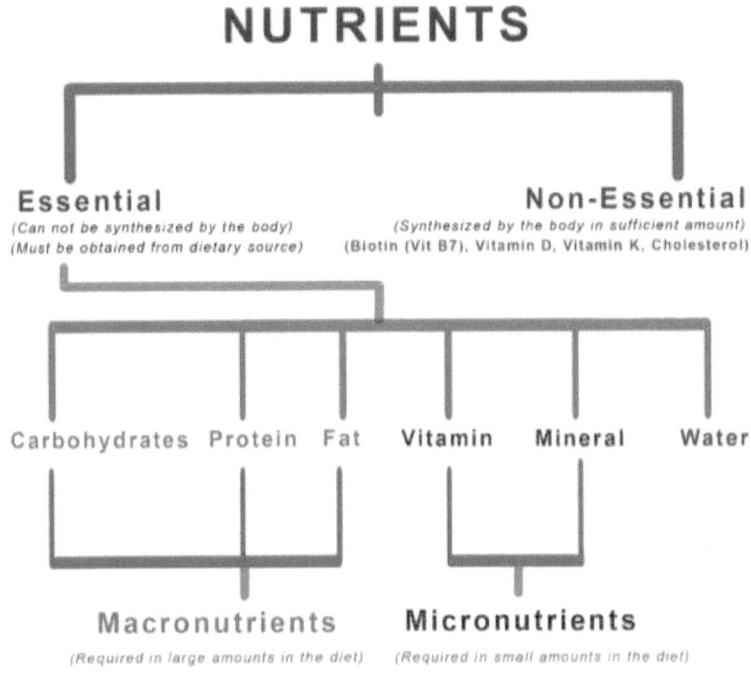

NUTRIENTS

Essential
(Can not be synthesized by the body)
(Must be obtained from dietary source)

Non-Essential
(Synthesized by the body in sufficient amount)
(Biotin (Vit B7), Vitamin D, Vitamin K, Cholesterol)

Carbohydrates Protein Fat Vitamin Mineral Water

Macronutrients
(Required in large amounts in the diet)

Micronutrients
(Required in small amounts in the diet)

©LaFonceur

Types of Nutrients:

Essential nutrients

Nonessential nutrients

ESSENTIAL NUTRIENTS

Essential nutrients either cannot be synthesized by the body or synthesized in insufficient quantity and are required for normal body functioning thus must be obtained from foods.

Essential nutrients are divided into 2 parts:

Macronutrients

Micronutrients

MACRONUTRIENTS

Macronutrients are the main nutrients that make up our foods. Body requires these nutrients in relatively large amounts to grow, develop, repair, and reproduce. They supply us with energy.

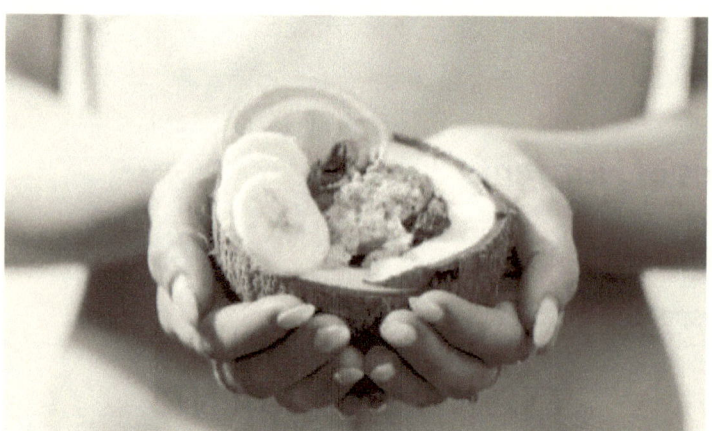

The three macronutrients are carbohydrate, protein, and fat, with the fourth bonus, water. All these three macronutrients have their specific functions in the body. Almost every food has all of the macronutrients, but foods are classified based on the highest percentage of macronutrient present in it. For example, a coconut consists up of 50% fat, 10% carbohydrates, and 6% protein, so this would be classified as fat, while a banana consists of 80% carbohydrates, with only small amounts of protein and fats, so this would be classified as a carbohydrate.

1. Carbohydrates

By definition, carbohydrates cannot be listed as essential macronutrients as the body can synthesize all the carbohydrates on its own, but it is recommended to get most of the energy from carbohydrates. Therefore, they are required in relatively large amounts for normal body functioning, and carbohydrates are a healthy nutrient choice.

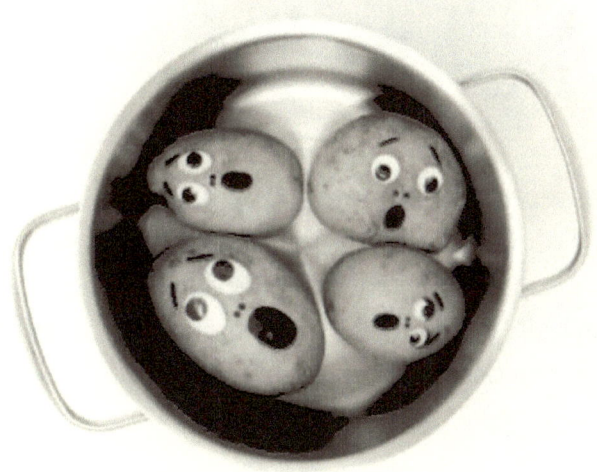

Carbohydrates are comprised of small chains of sugar that break down into glucose by enzyme salivary amylase present in our mouth to use as the body's primary energy source and therefore needs to make up around 50-65% of a diet. Carbohydrates are important in supplying energy to the brain, improving digestion, playing key roles in development, supporting normal immune function, preventing pathogenesis, and blood clotting.

2. Proteins

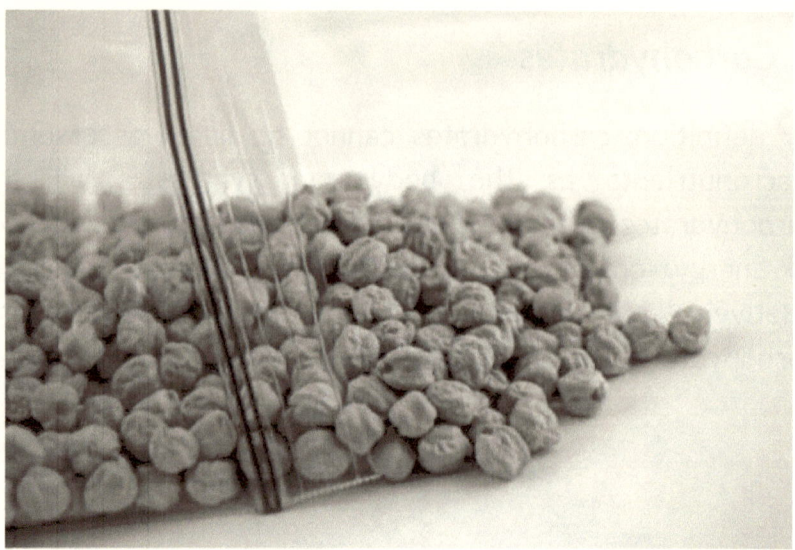

Proteins are essential macronutrients, consisting of one or more long chain of amino acid which is the essential part of all living organisms, especially as the building blocks of body tissue such as muscle, hair, bones, nails, etc. Among 20 amino acids, nine amino acids are essential which cannot be synthesized by the body.

Essential Proteins:

- Histidine

- Isoleucine

- Leucine

- Lysine

- Methionine

- Phenylalanine

- Threonine
- Tryptophan
- Valine

3. Fat

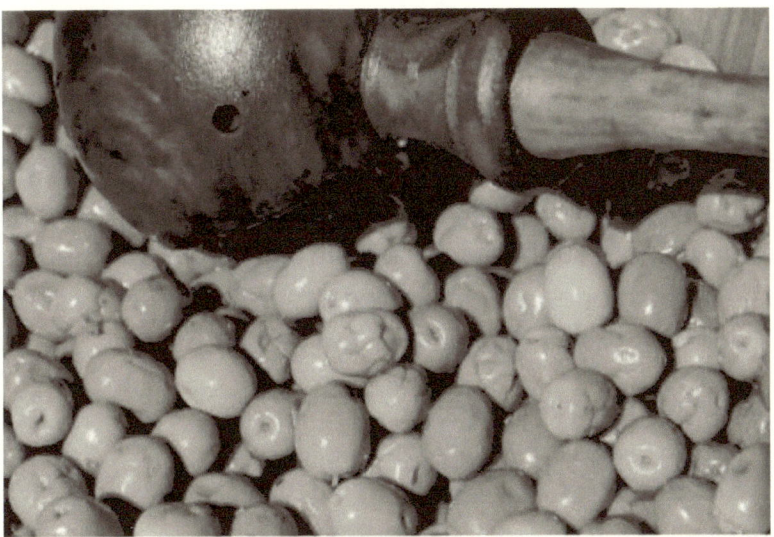

Fat is an essential nutrient and boosts absorption of fat-soluble vitamins such as Vitamin A, D, E, K and helps protect internal organs.

Essential Fatty acids:

- Alpha-linolenic acid (omega-3 fatty acid)
- Linoleic acid (omega-6 fatty acid)

MICRONUTRIENTS

Micronutrients are required in small amounts, but they are just as vital as macronutrients for normal body functioning. Micronutrients support metabolism and enable the body to produce hormones, enzymes, and other substances essential for proper growth and development.

Types of micronutrients:

Vitamins

Minerals

Vitamins

Vitamins are organic compounds. Humans require thirteen vitamins in their diet. Vitamins are classified as either water-soluble (vitamin B Complex and vitamin C) or fat-soluble (A, D, E, and K). Water-soluble vitamins get dissolve in water and are readily excreted from the body. This is why a consistent intake of water-soluble vitamins is required. Fat-soluble vitamins require lipid in the body to be absorbed through the intestinal tract.

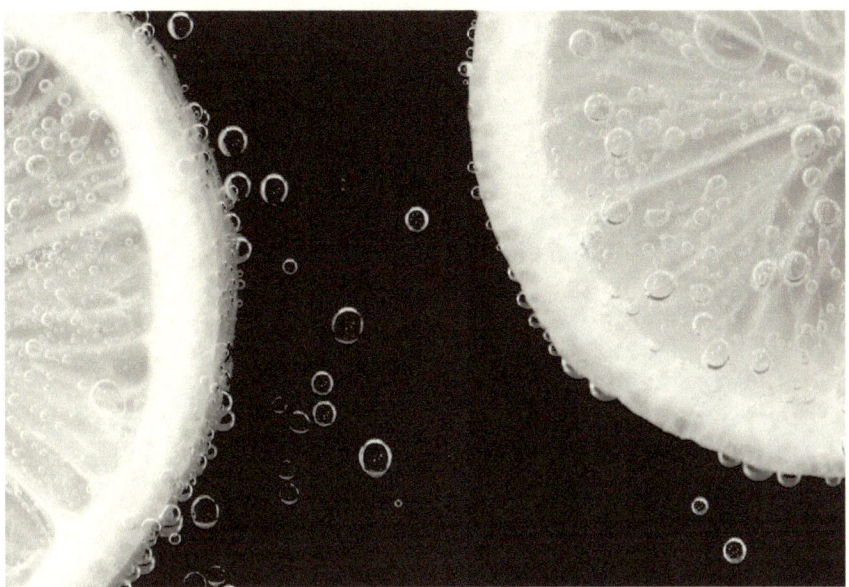

Vitamins are organic compounds. Humans require thirteen vitamins in their diet. Vitamins are classified as either water-soluble (vitamin B Complex and vitamin C) or fat-soluble (A, D, E, and K). Water-soluble vitamins get dissolve in water and are readily excreted from the body. This is why a consistent intake of water-soluble vitamins is required. Fat-soluble vitamins require lipid in the body to be absorbed through the intestinal tract.

Vitamins act as coenzymes or cofactors for various proteins, which are part of many chemical reactions in the body. Vitamin A is vital for healthy skin, teeth, mucus membranes, and eyes. Vitamin C for immunity. Vitamin D absorbs calcium to promote bone growth and cardiovascular health. Vitamin B6 helps form red blood cells and maintain brain function.

Essential Vitamins:

Fat-soluble vitamins

Water-soluble vitamins

Fat-soluble Vitamins are

- Vitamin A
- Vitamin D
- Vitamin E
- Vitamin K

Water-soluble Vitamins are

- Vitamin B Complex
  - Thiamine (Vitamin B1)
  - Riboflavin (Vitamin B2)
  - Niacin (Vitamin B3)
  - Pantothenic acid (Vitamin B5)
  - Pyroxidine (Vitamin B6)
  - Biotin (Vitamin B7)
  - Folate (Vitamin B9)
  - Cobalamin (Vitamin B12)
- Vitamin C

Vitamin B7 and Vitamin D can be synthesized by the body but in insufficient quantity.

Minerals

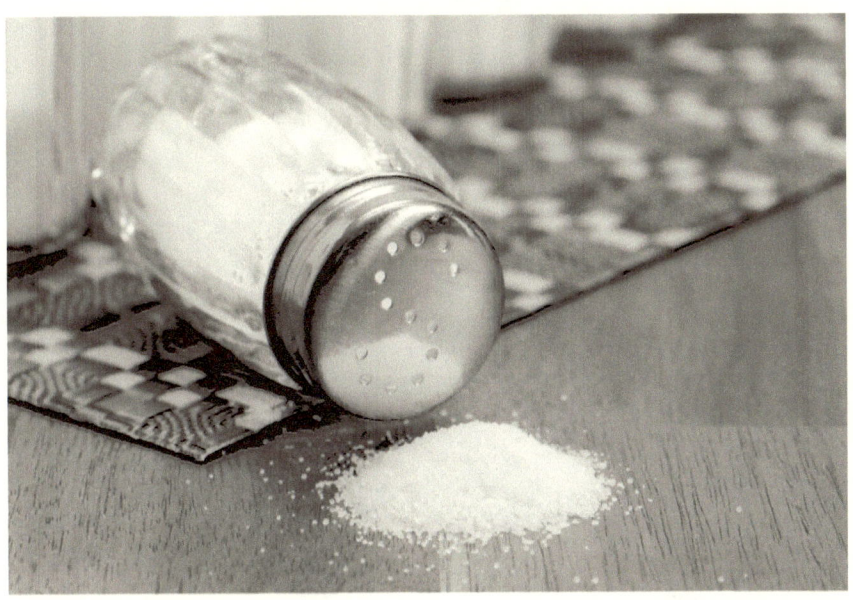

Minerals are inorganic and retain their chemical structure. Minerals are mainly needed for metabolism. They are important for healthy bones, muscle contraction, proper fluid balance, and nerve transmission in the body.

Essential Minerals:

Major Minerals

- Calcium

- Sodium

- Potassium

- Magnesium

- Phosphorus

Trace Minerals

- Iodine

- Iron

- Zinc

- Copper

- Chlorine

- Sulfur

- Manganese

- Cobalt

- Molybdenum

- Selenium

NONESSENTIAL NUTRIENTS

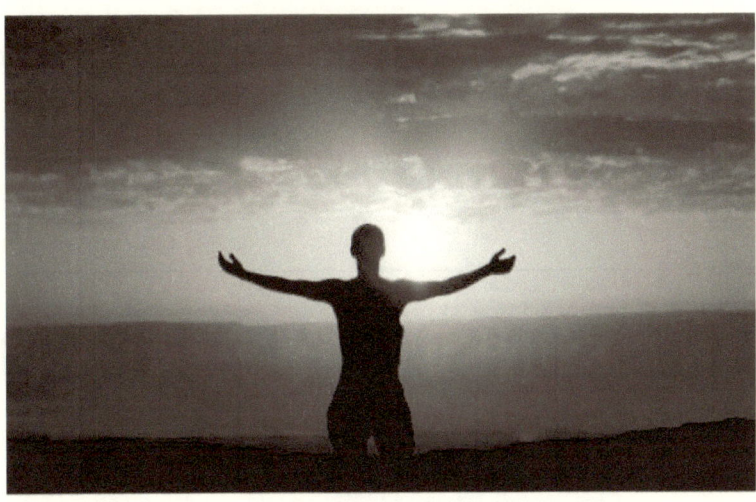

Nonessential nutrients can be synthesized by the body in sufficient quantity or obtained from sources other than foods.

Some examples of Nonessential nutrients:

- Biotin or Vitamin B7 is produced by gastrointestinal bacteria.

- Vitamin K is produced by intestinal bacteria present in the colon.

- Vitamin D is produced by the body when the skin is exposed to sunlight.

- Cholesterol is produced by the liver in a good amount. This is the reason you don't need to add extra cholesterol to your diet.

CHAPTER 2

10 REASONS WHY FAT IS NOT THE ENEMY. THE TRUTH ABOUT FATS!

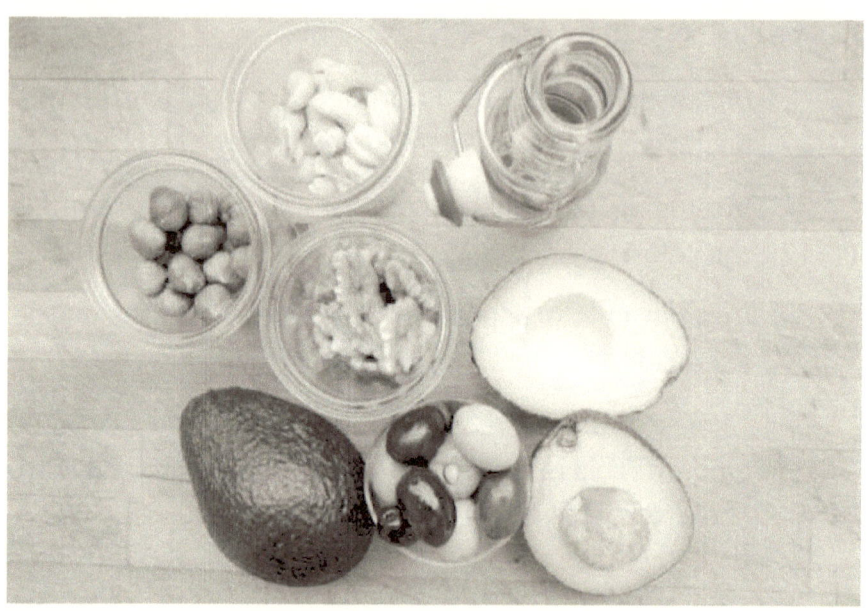

D id you know that the human brain is made up of nearly 60% fat? Fats are not something we should run from; our body needs a certain amount of fat to function at its best. Not all fats are bad, not all fats are good. Let's just quickly see which type of fat is our friend and which one is our enemy.

Types of fats:

Trans fats

Trans fats are the *worst* type of dietary fat. The hydrogenation process is used to turn healthy oils into solids to prevent them from becoming rancid, and a byproduct of this process is Trans fats. Trans fats have no known health benefits, and that there is no safe level of consumption. It is better to check the Nutritional Facts label on the packet of your packed food for any presence of trans fat. For every 2% of calories from trans-fat consumed daily, the risk of heart disease rises by 23%.

Food containing Trans Fat:

- Solid margarine
- French fries
- Vegetable shortening
- Pastries
- Cookies

Saturated Fats

They are solid at room temperature. A diet rich in saturated fats can increase total cholesterol, particularly harmful LDL cholesterol, that may cause blockages in arteries in the heart or elsewhere in the body. Saturated fat should be consumed in moderation, and it is recommended to limit the consumption of saturated fat to less than 10% calories a day.

Common sources of saturated fat:

- Whole milk
- Cheese
- Red meat
- Coconut oil
- Many commercially prepared baked goods

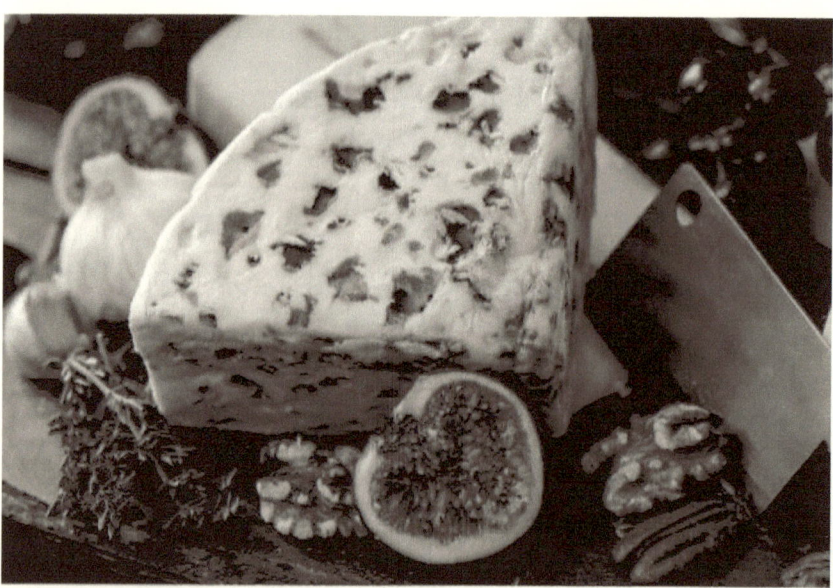

Unsaturated Fats

Monounsaturated and Polyunsaturated Fats

Monounsaturated and Polyunsaturated fats are healthy fats. They are liquid at room temperature and found in vegetables, nuts, and seeds. Polyunsaturated fats build cell membranes and the covering of nerves. They play an important role in blood clotting, muscle movement, and inflammation.

Good sources of monounsaturated fats are

- Extra virgin olive oil
- Sunflower oil
- Peanut oil
- Canola oil
- High-oleic safflower oil
- Avocado
- Nuts

Omega-3 fatty acids and omega-6 fatty acids are examples of polyunsaturated fats. Replacing saturated fats and refined carbohydrates with polyunsaturated fats can reduce harmful LDL cholesterol and improves the cholesterol profile. It also lowers triglycerides.

Good sources of omega-3 fatty acids include

- Flax seeds
- Chia seeds

- kidney beans

- Soybeans

- Walnut

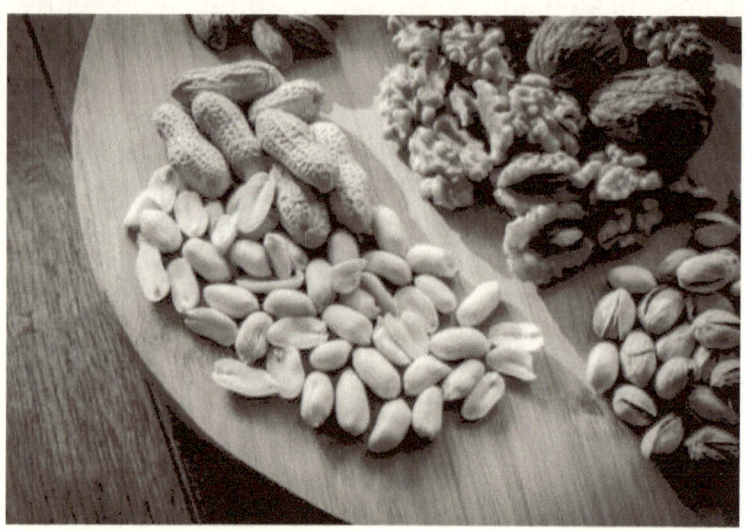

Omega-6 fatty acids have been linked to protection against heart disease.

Good sources of omega-6 fatty acids include

- Corn oil

- Sunflower oil

- Safflower oil

- Soybean oil

- Walnut

Below are the 10 reasons why fat is not the enemy:

1. Fat is Essential to Brain Health

Fat is essential to brain health. The brain is made of 60% fats, out of which a large chunk is docosahexaenoic acid (DHA) or Omega 3 fat.

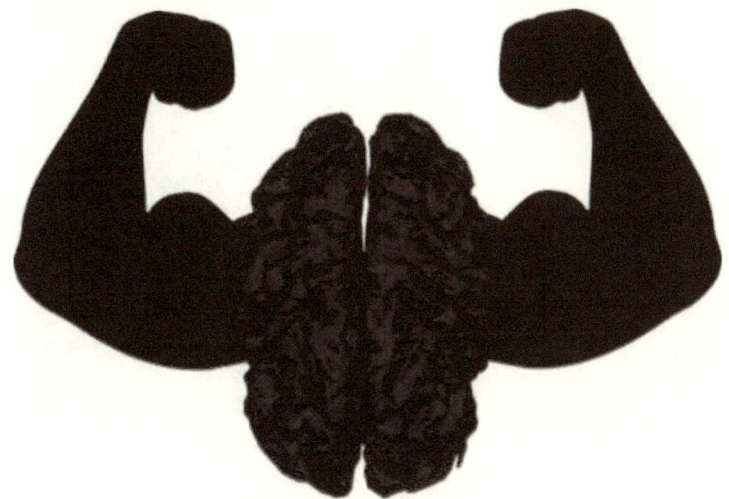

Essential fat-soluble vitamins such as A, D, E, and K are not water-soluble and require fat to get transported and absorbed in the body. These fat-soluble vitamins are crucial for brain health and many of our vital organs.

Vitamin D decreases susceptibility to Alzheimer's, Parkinson's, depression, and other brain disorders, and omega-3 is said to sharpen cognitive function and improve mood.

2. Fat for Better Skin

Fat makes up the bulk of the cellular membrane, and our skin is made up of a large number of cells. Without the proper consumption of fat, skin can become dry and chapped, which can also open up pathways for infection to enter our body.

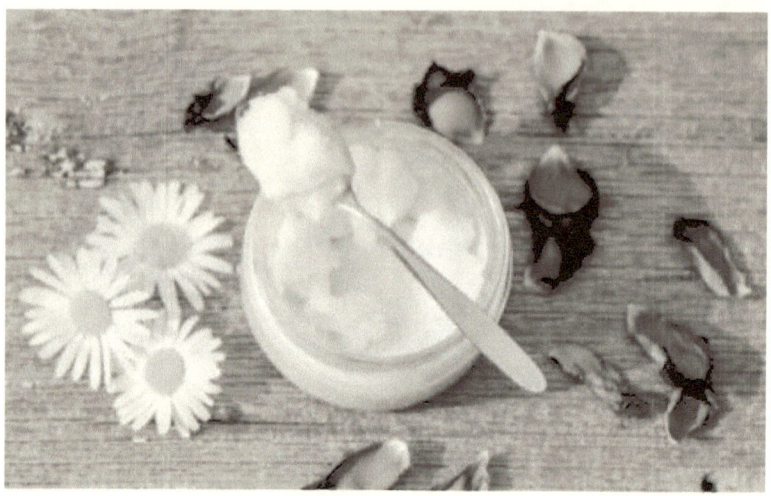

3. Fat Boosts Immune System

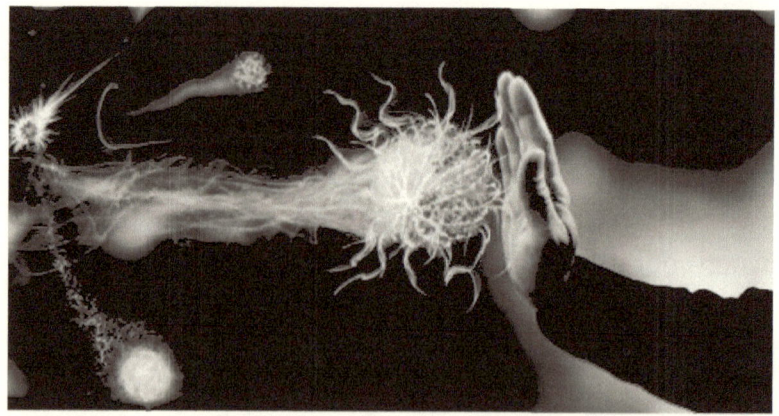

Fats are required for a healthy immune system. Saturated fats play an important role here, as adequate amounts will help the immune system recognize and then destroy foreign invaders.

Learn What are the Power Foods to Boost Your Immunity in the book Eat to Prevent and Controls Disease.

4. Fat Keeps Our Lungs Working Properly

Lungs are coated with a thin layer that is made up of 100% saturated fat. Fats are needed to protect this protective layer; Otherwise, it may result in breathing problems.

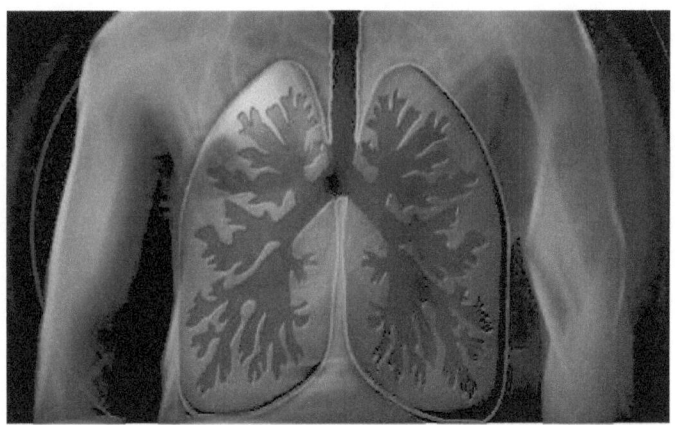

5. Fat is Good for Heart

Unsaturated fats are healthy for your heart because they help lower blood pressure and slows the build-up of plaque in arteries by reducing triglycerides, a type of fat in your blood. Switching from saturated fats to polyunsaturated or monounsaturated fats can lower heart disease risk by up to 25%.

6. Fat Can Help You Lose Weight (Yes, you read it right)

Hungry cells cause weight gain. When you limit your calorie intake, your body goes into starvation mode, holding onto calories and storing fat.

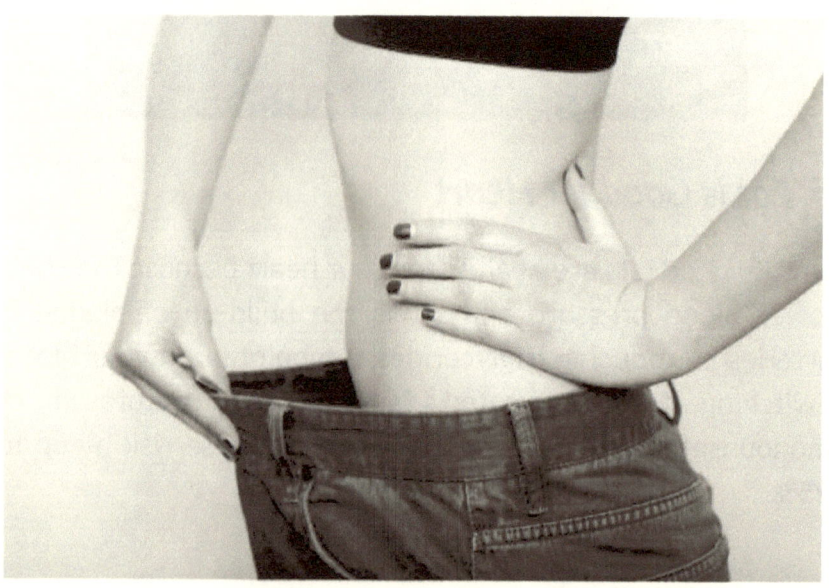

When you fuel your body with the right foods and enough healthy fats, your metabolism keeps running, and you are better at losing weight.

7. Fat for Proper Insulin Release

Saturated fats found in coconut oil help support proper nerve signaling by acting on signaling messengers. These messengers affect metabolism, as well as control the proper release of insulin.

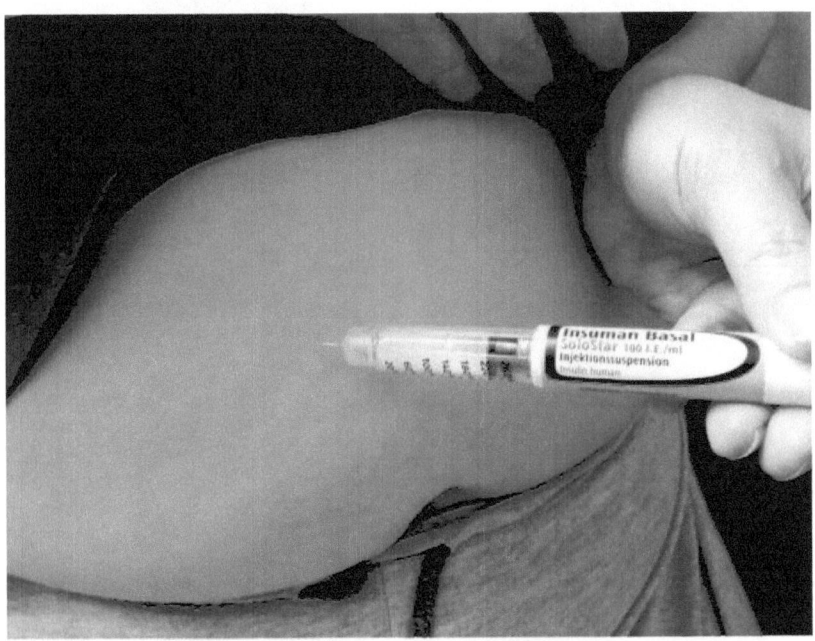

8. Fat for Stronger Bones and Less Risk of Osteoporosis

The important bone-building vitamins – Vitamin A, D, E, and K are only fat-soluble, which means they are transported and absorbed using dietary fats. Fat is required for the metabolism of calcium.

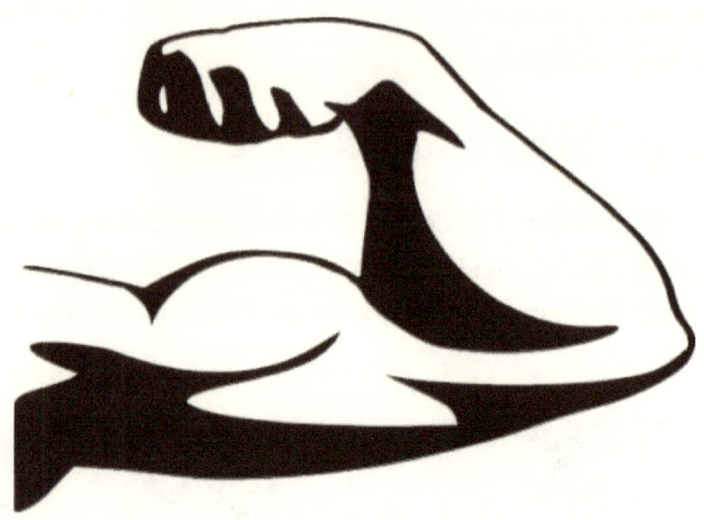

9. Fat for Better Reproductive Health

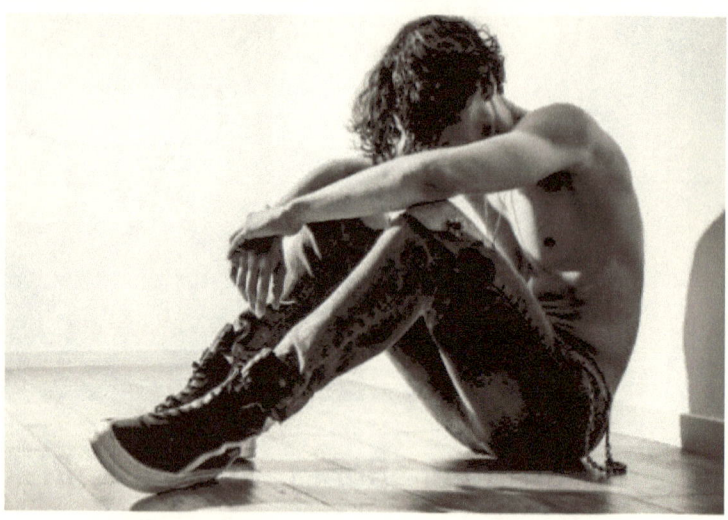

Fats are the building blocks for healthy cell membranes and are important for hormonal health. Sex hormones – testosterone, estrogen, progesterone – are all made of cholesterol. Cutting way back on dietary fats can increase your risk of hormonal problems like hypothyroidism, menstrual irregularities, and low testosterone levels for men.

10. Fat for Better Eye Health

In dry eye disease, lack of tears leads to dryness, discomfort, and occasional blurry vision. Omega-3 fats help produce more tears and may benefit people with this condition. In addition, omega-3 fats help prevent diabetic retinopathy due to their anti-inflammatory properties.

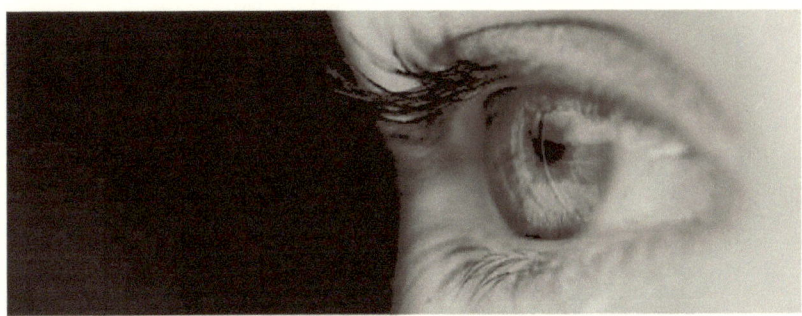

Conclusion

No doubt not all fats are good for health, but at the same time, certain types of fats are essential for our health. Try to eat monounsaturated and polyunsaturated fats as much as you can (not beyond the limit) and limit your saturated fat consumption to less than 10%. Try replacing butter with extra virgin olive oil and French fries with nuts. These small changes in diet will result in a healthier and longer life.

CHAPTER 3

TOP 10 HEALTHY FAT FOODS YOU SHOULD EAT

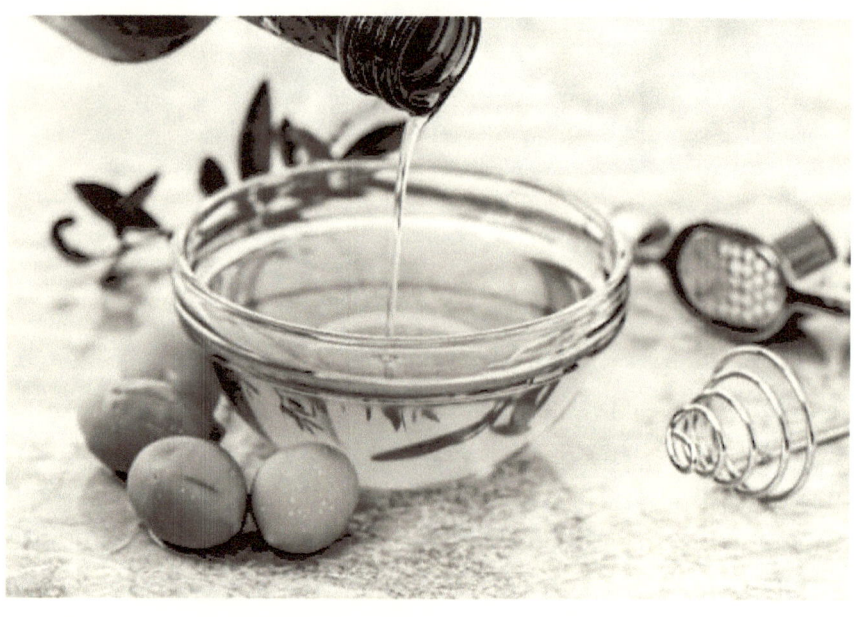

From decades fat is associated with weight gain, heart diseases, and many more. But now is the time you understand all types of fats are not the devil. If you avoid fats but have no control over sugar, processed and refined carbs consumption, it is more dangerous to your health. Fat not only stores energy but insulates and protects vital organs. In fact, healthy fats boost your heart health, improve cholesterol levels and enhance your beauty by making your skin glowing and hair shiny.

Focus more on foods rich in unsaturated fats (monounsaturated and polyunsaturated) but don't 100% avoid saturated fats.

Below I have listed the top 10 healthy fat sources you should eat for health and nutritional benefits.

1. Ghee

Ghee is a form of clarified butter. It is generally used in Indian cooking. Ghee made from cow milk has immense health benefits as per Ayurved. Cow ghee is full of essential nutrients, fatty acids, antioxidants. It has antibacterial, anti-fungal, and antiviral properties. Ghee is rich in conjugated linoleic acid, or CLA, a fatty acid known to protect against carcinogens, diabetes, and artery plaque. It is known as a brain tonic and excellent for improving memory power and intelligence. It is beneficial for curing thyroid dysfunction. It heals wounds, chapped lips, and mouth ulcers. It also cures insomnia and is best for the lubrication of joints.

Ghee has a high smoke point which means ghee doesn't go rancid even at high temperature and retains all the important nutrients that provide all the incredible ghee benefits. Ghee is a rich source of vitamin A, vitamin E, and vitamin K, keeping your skin glowing and maintaining healthy vision. Vitamin K found in ghee helps prevent calcium deposits in the arteries that can obstruct blood flow and lead to blockages. Ghee should consume in moderation if you don't want to put on weight. 1 tablespoon (15g) of ghee in a day is enough to ripe all the health benefits of ghee.

2. Extra Virgin Olive Oil

Extra virgin olive oil is one of the world's healthiest oils. Eating about 2 tablespoons of extra virgin olive oil every day may reduce the risk of coronary heart disease due to the presence of monounsaturated fats in olive oil. Extra virgin olive oil is loaded with powerful antioxidants that inhibit oxidation and prevent the formation of free radicals in the body, which reduce the risk of chronic diseases and cancer.

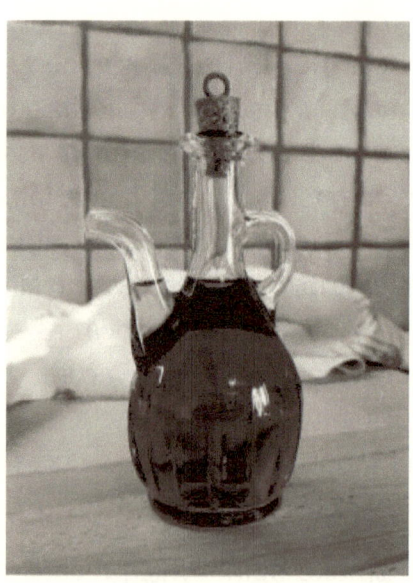

Do not use extra virgin olive oil for cooking at high temperatures, such as deep-frying, as it oxidizes quicker than other oils.

3. Coconut & Coconut Oil

Lauric acid is why coconut is considered healthy, even though it contains almost 89% of saturated fats. Lauric acid, a 12-carbon atom chain, is a saturated fatty acid found in coconut with antibacterial, antiviral, and antimicrobial properties that prevent infections. Coconut oil is good for your skin and hair.

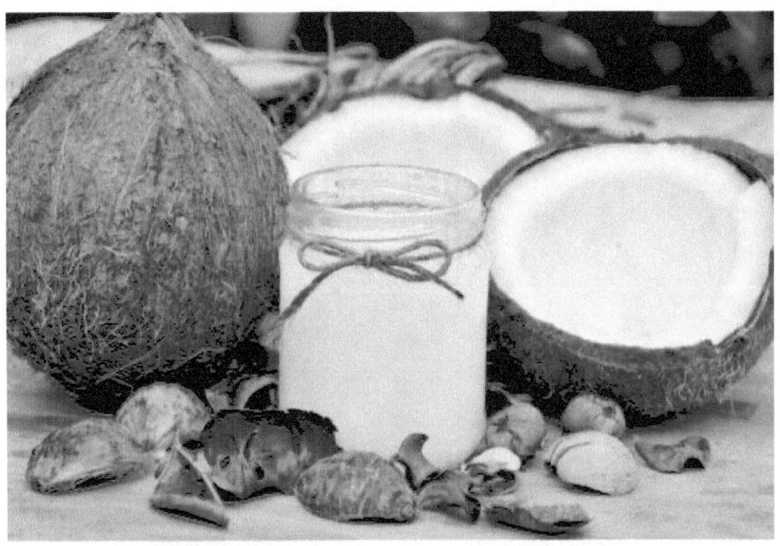

Coconut oil has anti-inflammatory properties due to antioxidants present in it, potentially helping to reduce arthritis symptoms. Saturated fat in coconut oil increases HDL levels (good cholesterol) and promotes heart health, but at the same time, it increases LDL levels (bad cholesterol) too; therefore, it should be consumed in moderation.

Read Top 10 Foods that Prevent Hair Loss and Promote Hair Growth in the book Secret of Healthy Hair.

4. Avocado

Avocado is loaded with vitamin B complex, vitamin K, vitamin C, and vitamin E. It is also rich in phytosterols and carotenoids such as lutein and zeaxanthin. These carotenoids are converted into vitamin A in the body and protect the eyes from diseases by absorbing harmful blue light entering the eyes. Vitamin K in avocado can support bone health by increasing calcium absorption.

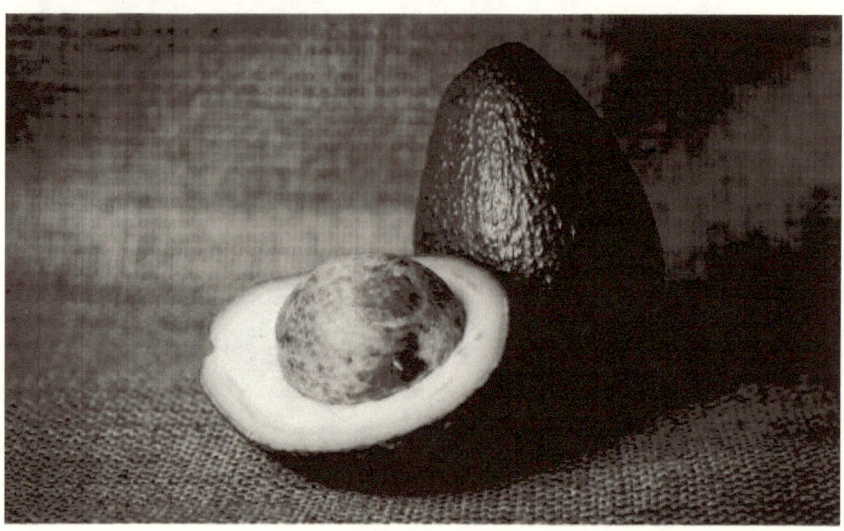

Dietary fiber in avocado improves digestion. About 75% of an avocado's calories come from fat, mostly monounsaturated fats MUFAs (about 65%) like oleic acid and linoleic acid. These monounsaturated fats are strongly associated with reduced risks of developing diabetes, heart disease, and high blood pressure.

5. Flaxseeds

Flaxseeds are high in unsaturated omega-3 fatty acids: alpha-linolenic acid (ALA), which protects against heart disease by improving blood pressure. Only 1-2 tablespoons of Flaxseeds are enough to reap the benefits.

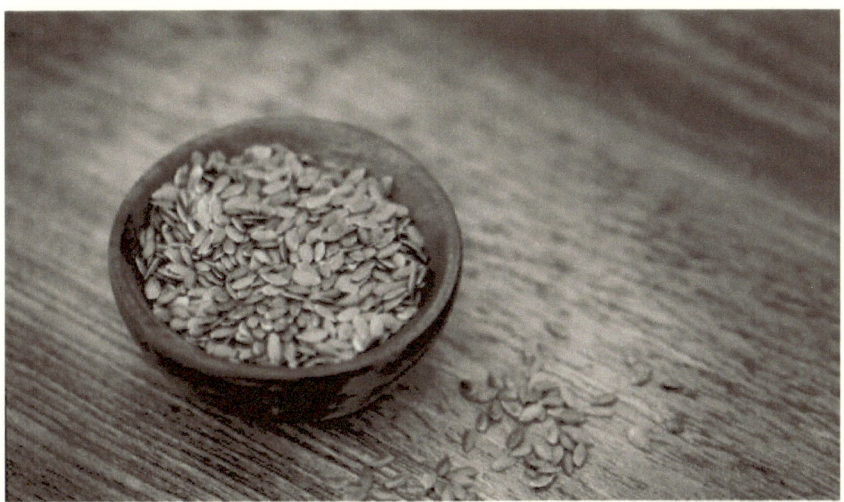

Flaxseed contains both soluble and insoluble fiber that leaves you feeling full for a long time, reducing weight as well as lowering cholesterol levels. Regular intake of flaxseeds is good for your skin and heart. Flaxseeds contain other nutrients such as protein, magnesium, calcium, phosphorus, omega-3, and lignin. Lignans in flaxseed have antioxidant and estrogen properties that prevent cancer.

6. Black Sesame Seeds

Black sesame seeds are high in unsaturated fatty acids while low in saturated fatty acids. Black sesame is considered one of the best anti-aging foods according to traditional Chinese medicine. Sesame seeds are high in calcium, copper, and magnesium, which are bone-forming minerals.

The oleic acid and linoleic acid in black sesame seeds promote skin softening and cell regeneration, improving skin health. The higher iron content of black sesame seeds helps in preventing iron-deficiency anemia.

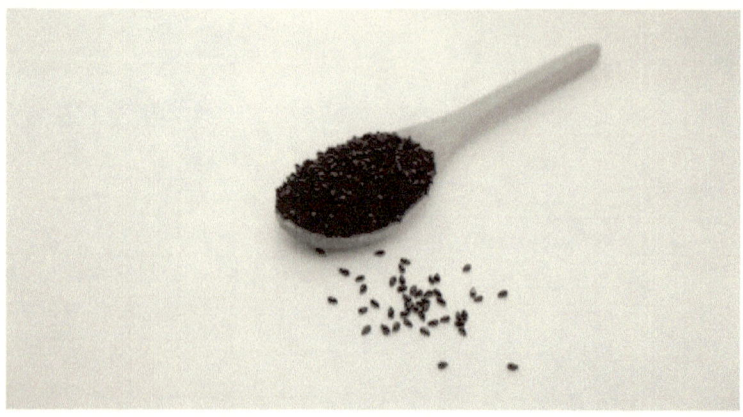

7. Walnuts

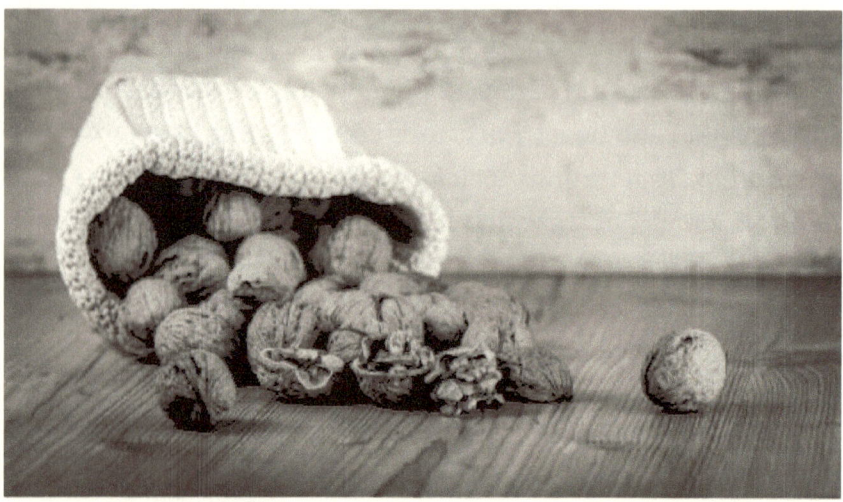

Unlike most nuts, walnuts are high in polyunsaturated fatty

acids - omega-3 fats, especially alpha-linolenic acid (ALA), linoleic acid, and oleic acid, which protects against heart disease.

Eat walnuts for better brain function and better memory. Walnuts may help lower blood pressure. The anti-inflammatory property of walnut reduces the risk of breast and prostate cancers. Antioxidants in walnut are of higher quality and potency than any other nut.

8. Almonds

Almonds contain high levels of monounsaturated and polyunsaturated fats and have a significant positive impact on cholesterol levels.

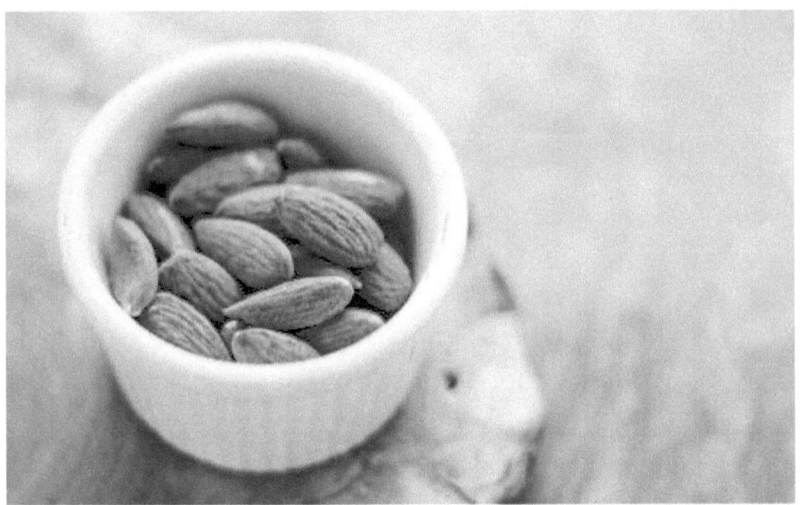

The protein and fiber content of almonds make them the best option for snack because a handful of almonds can satisfy you for at least a few hours, increasing your chances of losing weight successfully. Biotin (also known as vitamin H) in almonds improves hair health. Almonds are rich in vitamin E and antioxidants, which improve skin health.

9. Dark chocolate

Dark chocolate is rich in flavanols, a powerful antioxidant that can lower blood pressure and allow more blood to flow to the heart, therefore improving heart health. Although half of the dark chocolate fat content is saturated fats, it is a good source of vitamins A, B, and E, iron, calcium, potassium, magnesium.

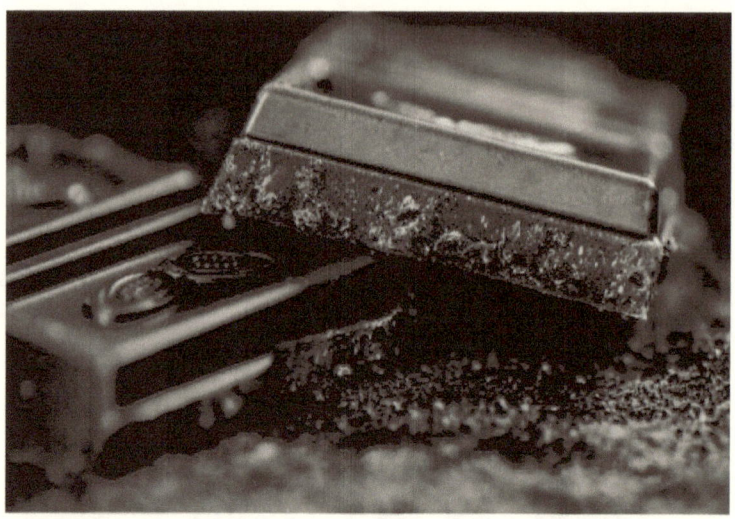

Also, dark chocolate helps improve cognitive performance but make sure you eat chocolate with 70 percent cocoa for the highest flavonoids and avoid milk chocolate, which contains loads of sugar and dairy.

10. Dairy

Cow's milk is good for the bones because it is a rich source of calcium, an essential mineral for healthy bones and teeth. Cow's milk is a good source of potassium, which can reduce blood pressure, and risk of cardiovascular disease.

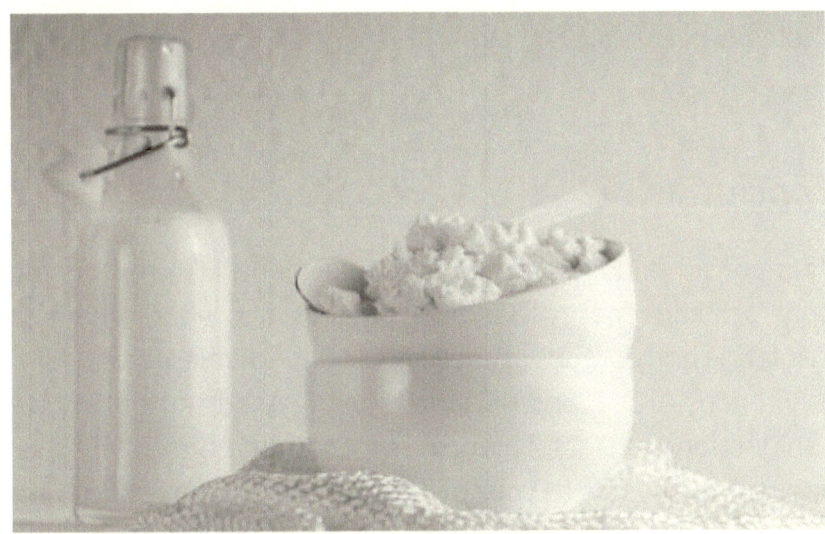

Some available **Cheese** options are healthy as they fulfill the body's calcium and potassium need. Cottage cheese, feta, ricotta are the top healthiest cheese options available.

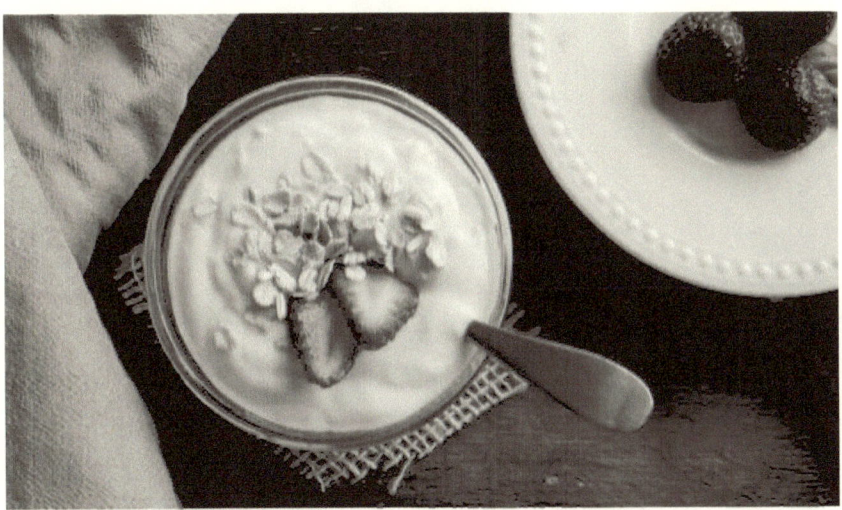

Probiotic yogurt helps keep the intestine healthy and strengthen the digestive tract. Probiotic yogurt increases the good bacteria in your gut to promote better overall health. Daily intake of probiotic yogurt boosts immunity and reduces cholesterol levels.

Conclusion

Fats are an important dietary requirement. Healthy fats not only provide energy but also protect our vital organs by insulating body organs against shock. Fat-soluble vitamins such as vitamins A, D, E, and K can only be digested and absorbed in conjunction with fats. This proves fats are not the enemy. Start adding healthy fats to your diet from today. Happy eating.

CHAPTER 4

TOP 10 FOODS FOR VEGETARIANS TO PREVENT VITAMIN B12 DEFICIENCY

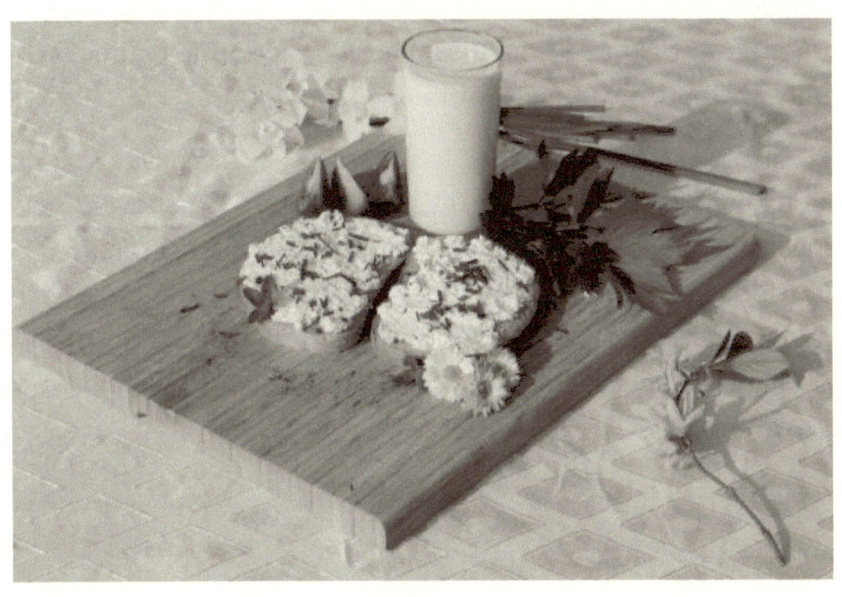

f you feel fatigued, depressed, and irritated all the time. If you hear a ringing sound in 1 or both ears or experiencing memory trouble and poor balance, you may have Vitamin B12 Deficiency, also known as Cobalamin Deficiency. Protein foods are the primary sources of vitamin B12, including animal meats and fish, which is why vegetarians often lack vitamin B12.

What is Vitamin B12 and Why is it Important?

Vitamin B12 or cobalamin is a water-soluble vitamin. It is an essential nutrient important in the nervous system's normal functioning, helps make DNA, the genetic material in human cells, and keeps blood cells healthy. Vitamin B12 deficiency may lead to a reduction in healthy red blood cells that may result in anemia. The Dietary Reference Intake (DRI), for adult men and women, is 2.4 micrograms of vitamin B12 in a day. Like other essential nutrients, Vitamin B12 cannot be made by the body. Instead, it should be obtained from food.

If your vitamin B12 level is quite low, you have to take supplements or vitamin B12 injections, whichever your physician advises. But if you have borderline vitamin B12 deficiency or want to prevent it in the future, you must start eating vitamin B12 rich foods. Although vitamin B12 is mainly found in animal sources, there are some vegetarian options to prevent its deficiency.

I am listing below the top 10 vitamin B12 rich foods for vegetarians.

1. Yogurt

Eating yogurt daily is an excellent way to get more vitamin B12. Yogurt has the highest absorption of vitamin B12, between 50% and 75%. Yogurt is also a good source of folate and vitamin B6. Go for low-fat, unsweetened plain yogurt to avoid weight gain.

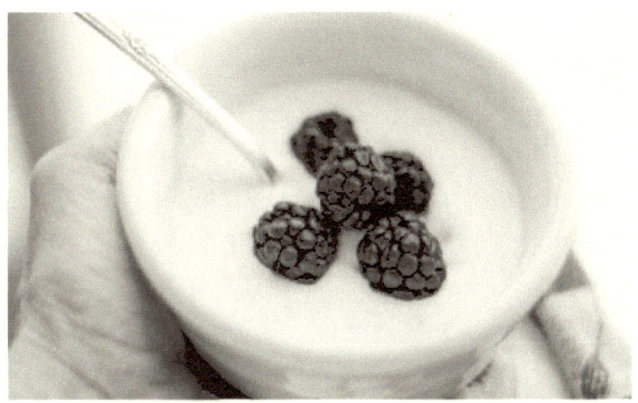

2. Cow's Milk

Milk is another excellent source of vitamin B12, and adequate consumption may help prevent the vitamin B12 deficiency. About 2 cups of 250 ml of milk per day can get you the recommended daily intake of vitamin B12. It is loaded with other nutrients such as calcium, protein, potassium, and phosphorus. Have it with breakfast cereal, and you will get more Vitamin B12.

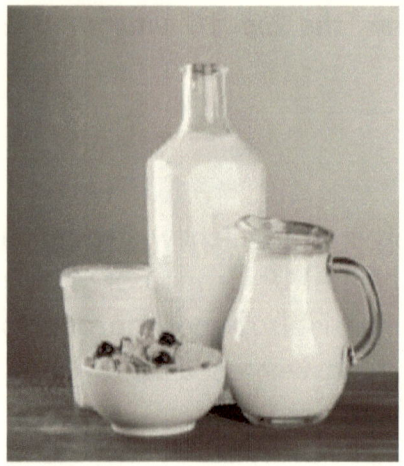

3. Cheese

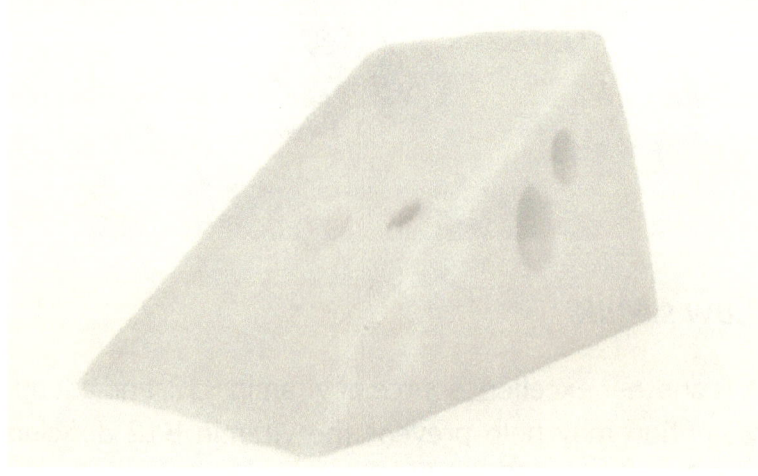

Cheese is a good source of vitamin B12. Some types of cheese, such as Swiss cheese, mozzarella cheese, and cottage cheese, are high in vitamin B12. Avoid processed cheese as the amount of vitamin B12 is very low in it. 1 slice of cheese is enough to provide you 22% to 36% of the recommended daily intake of vitamin B12 but do not solely depend upon cheese to fulfill your daily vitamin B12 requirement as large consumption of cheese may make you fat.

4. Soy Milk

As such, soy milk does not naturally contain vitamin B12, but it can be fortified with it. Fortified food means that food has added nutrients that do not naturally occur in that food. In the case of soy milk, it is often fortified with vitamin B12 - be sure to check the label. Avoid flavored ones and choose unsweetened varieties as they are more natural and free of void calories, that is, sugar. With just one cup of fortified soy milk, you can get a day's worth of vitamin B12 (2.4 micrograms).

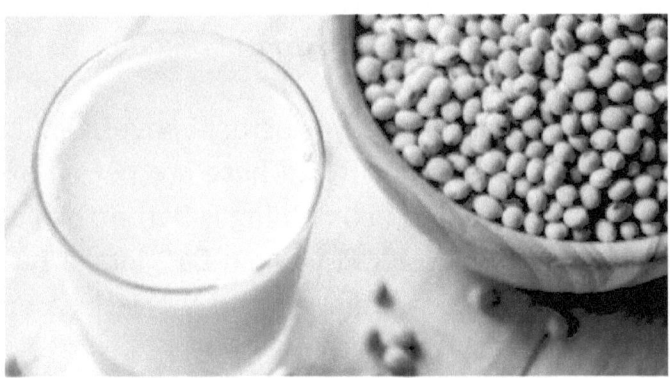

5. Tempeh

Tempeh is made by a culturing and controlled fermentation process that binds soybeans into a cake form. Bacterial contamination during tempeh production may contribute to the increased vitamin B12 content of tempeh. The amount of vitamin B12 present in tempeh is relatively low in comparison to milk products. Therefore, you shouldn't solely rely on it to meet your daily recommended vitamin B12 requirement. Still, it can boost your plant-based protein intake, giving you plenty of fiber with no cholesterol or saturated fat.

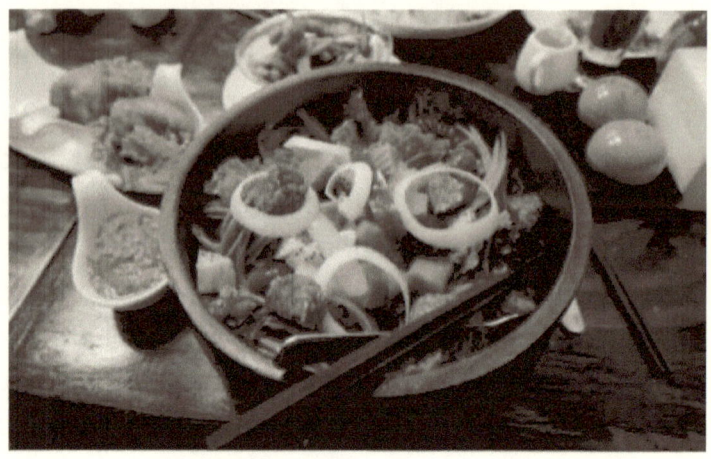

6. Dried Shiitake mushroom

Dried Shiitake Mushrooms, a type of fungi, have been shown to contain significant levels of B12. These are not an excellent source of vitamin B12, but something is better than nothing. You can increase your overall vitamin B12 intake by adding dried shiitake mushrooms, tempeh, and cheese in your wraps and stuffing.

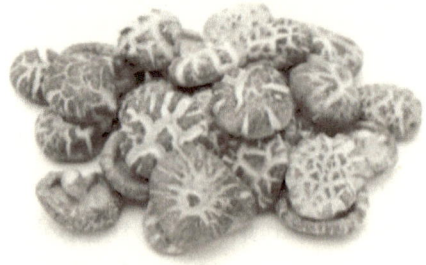

7. Whey Protein

Whey protein is a great source of vitamin B12. You can make

your own whey protein at home by curdling boiled milk with lemon juice. The liquid part of this process is your whey, which is rich in vitamin B12 and a great source of protein for vegetarians. Use this whey in your pancake batter or add it to your pasta recipes to get the full health benefits of whey.

8. Cereal

Breakfast cereal such as muesli and granola is a good source of vitamin B12. If you don't enjoy your cereal with milk, eat cereal as a snack during office break time or try it as a late-night snack. Be sure to go for unsweetened varieties to avoid unnecessary fat in your diet.

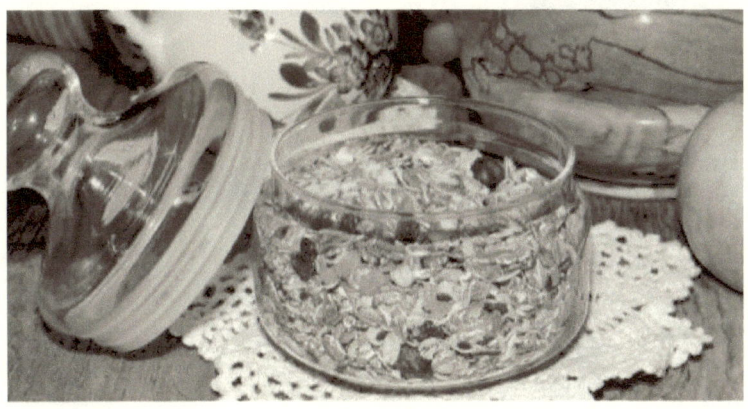

9. Vanilla Ice Cream

Ice cream is made of milk, and vitamin B12 is naturally found in milk, making ice cream a good source of vitamin B12. Not only this, but ice cream also contains vitamin A, B complex, C, D, K, and E, calcium, and protein. On the other hand, it is high in cholesterol and saturated fat. Therefore, it should be consumed in a lesser amount for overall health. A single cup serving of vanilla ice cream contains 20 percent of the recommended daily intake of vitamin B12.

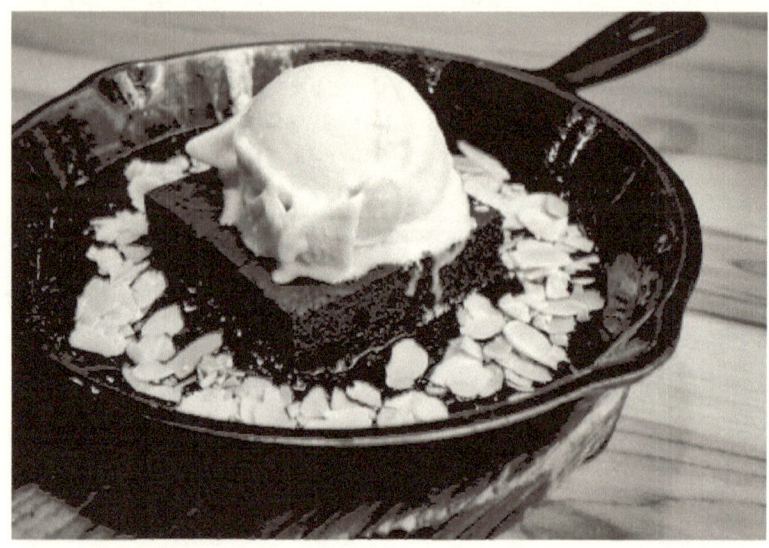

10. Rice Milk

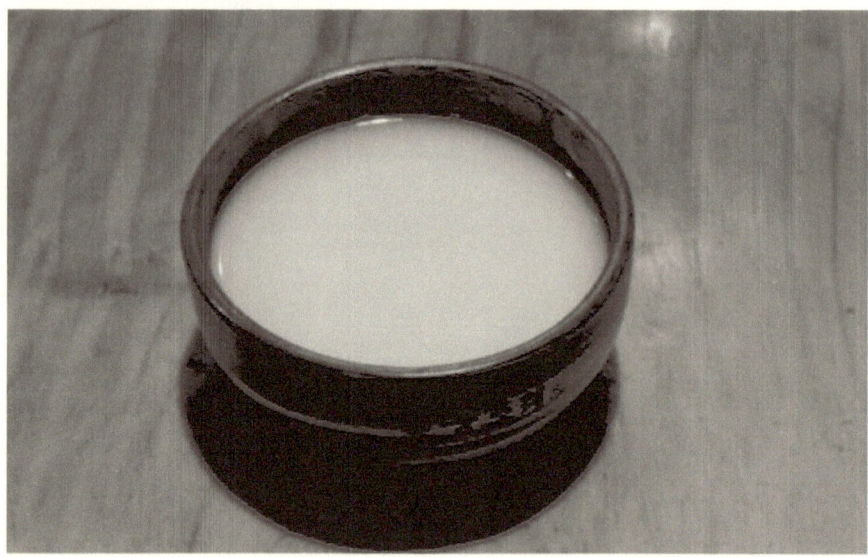

Rice milk is a good source of vitamin B12. It has zero saturated fat and rich in vitamin A, D, calcium, magnesium, potassium, and iron. You can make it at your home by finely blending a ½ cup of cooked brown rice with 2 cups of water. For extra smooth rice milk, simply pass the liquid through the strainer to remove any lumps. It tastes best when served chilled.

Conclusion

Vitamin B12 deficiency is not very uncommon among vegetarians, but all you have to do is make some little changes to your diet or, more accurately, include more vitamin B12 rich foods in your diet. With a few simple changes, you can have great results. It will not only prevent vitamin B12 deficiency, but it will also prevent anemia. Since vitamin B12 foods are rich in protein, you will get the double benefit of a healthy nervous system, healthy skin, and many more.

CHAPTER 5

RECIPES

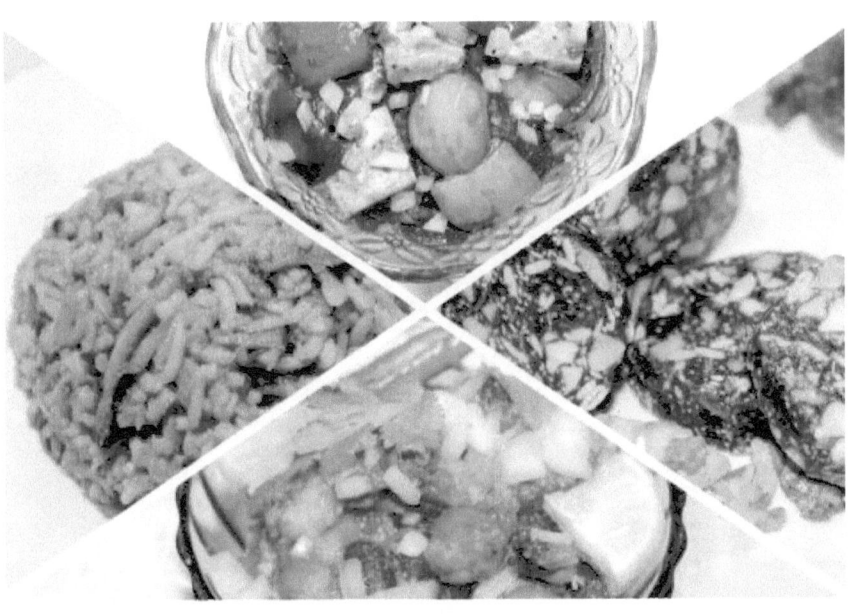

Chilli Tofu

Beans in Schezwan Sauce

Mushroom Fried Pulao

Khajur Roll

Chilli Tofu

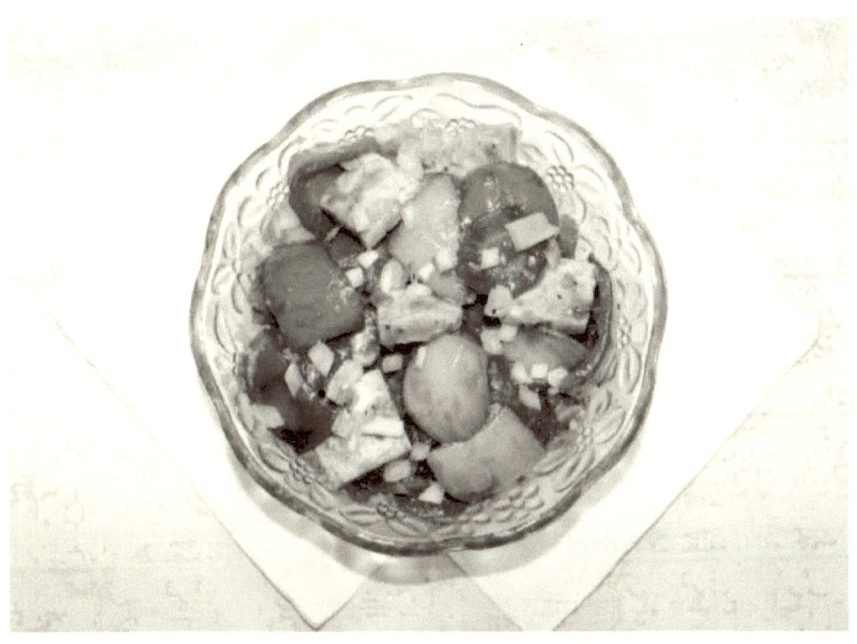

<u>Serves 2</u>

Ingredients

Tofu: 100 gm

Capsicum: 100 gm

Carrot: 100 gm

Onion: 100 gm

Chopped garlic: 2 tablespoons

Chopped ginger: 1 teaspoon

Red chili sauce: 1 tablespoon

Soy sauce: 1 tablespoon

Tomato sauce: 1 tablespoon

White Sesame seeds: 1 teaspoon

Black pepper powder: ½ teaspoon

Dry mango powder: 1 teaspoon (optional)

Vinegar: 1 teaspoon

Corn flour: 1 tablespoon

Salt to Taste

Water: 50 ml + 2 tablespoons (if required)

Mustard oil: 2 tablespoons

Spring onion: To garnish

Method

1. Cut tofu into 1-inch cubes and sprinkle some salt and pepper over it.

2. Chop capsicum, carrot, and onion in 1-inch cubes.

3. Mix 1 tablespoon of cornflour in 50 ml of water and keep aside.

4. In a bowl, mix soy sauce, red chili sauce, and tomato sauce. Keep aside.

5. Heat mustard oil in a pan. Add sesame seeds. Once splutter, add chopped ginger and garlic.

6. Now turn the flame to high. Cook for 1-2 min. Keep the flame

on high for the rest of the steps.

7. Add capsicum and cook for 2 to 3 min and then add carrot and cook for 2-3 min. Gradually mix so that veggies cook evenly. Don't overcook. Veggies should be crisp and crunchy, not soggy.

8. Add onion. Cook on high flame for 3-4 min or till it becomes slightly translucent. Do not overcook otherwise it will become soggy.

9. Turn the flame to low and add sauce mix. Add black pepper, salt, and ½ teaspoon dry mango powder or vinegar. Mix well.

10. Add the cornflour paste and turn the flame to high. Once it starts boiling and the sauce become thick, add tofu pieces. Mix well. Cook for another 2 -3 min till tofu absorbs all the flavors.

11. Turn off the flame. Take it into a bowl and sprinkle some dry mango powder. Garnish with spring onion and enjoy it while it still hot.

Note: As MSG (Monosodium glutamate) is not a healthy option, it is not added to this recipe. You can replace mustard oil with any other oil if it is not available to you. Adding dry mango powder is optional. We are using mustard oil and dry mango powder combination to have a similar taste as MSG.

Beans in Schezwan Sauce

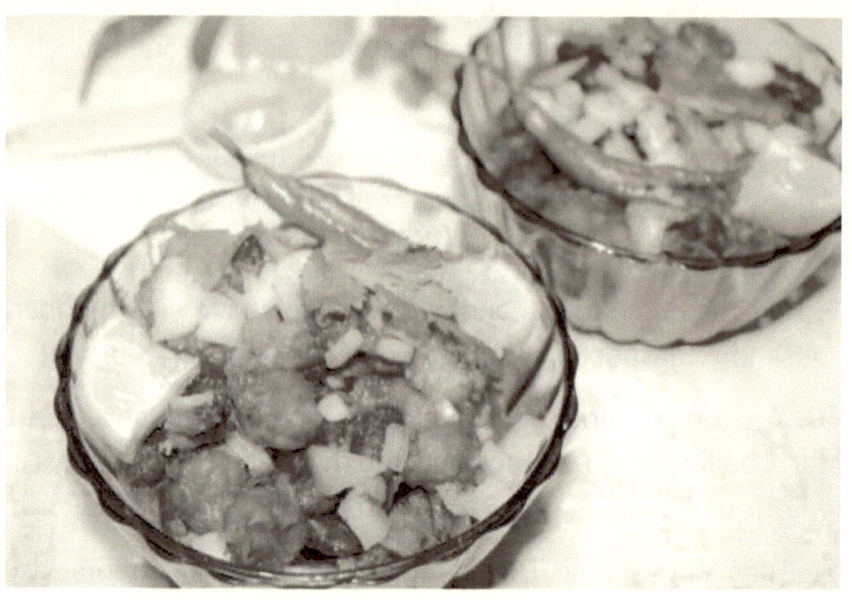

<u>Serves 2</u>

Ingredients:

Boiled chickpeas: 1½ cup

Boiled kidney beans: ½ cup

Boiled potatoes: 1 medium

Onion: 1 medium

Cumin: 1 teaspoon

Salt to Taste

Chopped garlic: 2 tablespoons

Chopped ginger: 1 tablespoon

Schezwan sauce: 2 tablespoons

Coriander leaves: To garnish

Green chilies: To garnish

Lemon: To garnish

Chopped onion: To garnish

Oil: 1 tablespoon

Method:

1. Heat oil in a pan. Add cumin. Sauté for 2 mins.

2. Add garlic and ginger. Cook for 2 mins on high flame.

3. Add chopped onion and cook till it becomes translucent.

4. Add chickpeas and kidney beans. Cook for 2 mins.

5. Add schezwan sauce and salt. Mix well.

6. Add chopped boiled potatoes. Cook on high for 2 mins.

7. Add 2 tablespoons of water if it looks dry. Cook for 5 mins on low to medium flame.

8. Turn off the flame. Garnish with chopped onion, coriander leaves, green chilies, and lemon. Enjoy beans in schezwan sauce with evening tea.

Mushroom Fried Pulao

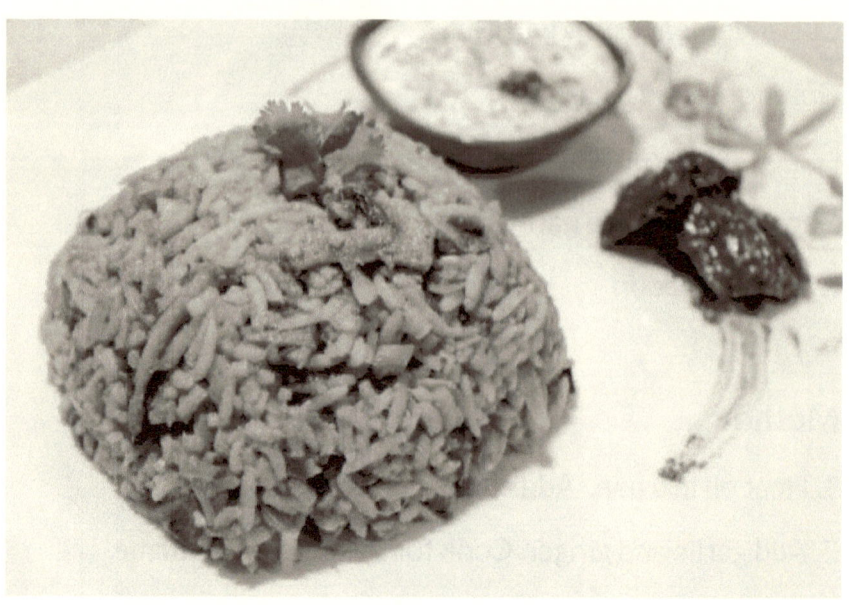

<u>**Serves: 2**</u>

Ingredients:

Mushroom: 100 gm

Cooked brown rice: 2 cups

Cumin: 1 tablespoon

Asafoetida: a pinch

Cashew nuts: 5 broken

Raisins: 8-10

Onion: 2 medium size

Chopped Garlic: 2 tablespoons

Tomatoes: 2 medium size

Yogurt: 2 tablespoons

Salt to Taste

Turmeric powder: 1 teaspoon

Coriander-cumin powder: 1 teaspoon

Garam masala: 1 teaspoon

Oil: 2 tablespoons

Method:

1. Warm oil in a pan. Add cashew nuts and fry till golden brown. Remove cashew nuts from oil.

2. Add asafetida and cumin to the remaining oil. Cook for a min.

3. Add garlic and cook for a min. Don't burn the garlic. Add onion and cook for about 5 mins on low to medium flame or till it becomes translucent.

4. Add tomatoes and salt. Salt will soften the tomatoes faster. Cover with a lid and cook for about 10-15 mins at low flame. Tomatoes should be softened completely. Mash the tomatoes with a spatula.

5. Add turmeric, coriander-cumin powder, red chili powder, and garam masala. Mix well. If it looks dry, add 2 -3 tablespoons of water. Cover with lid and cook for 5 mins or till it leaves oil. Few drops of oil will be visible on the sides of the tomato mix.

6. Add chopped mushrooms. Mix well and cover it with a lid. Let the mushrooms absorb all the spices.

7. Turn the flame to low and add yogurt. Mix for 2 mins. Add cooked brown rice and mix gently. Cook on medium-high flame for 5 mins.

8. Add cashew nuts and raisins. Mix well.

9. Turn off the flame, sprinkle coriander leaves and cover with a lid and leave for 10 mins.

10. Now it is ready to serve. Enjoy mushroom fried pulao with curd and pickle.

Note: Whenever using brown rice, always leave the dish covered for at least 10 mins. Brown rice absorbs flavors slowly as compared to white rice. Covering ensure the flavor to lock in the brown rice.

Khajur Roll

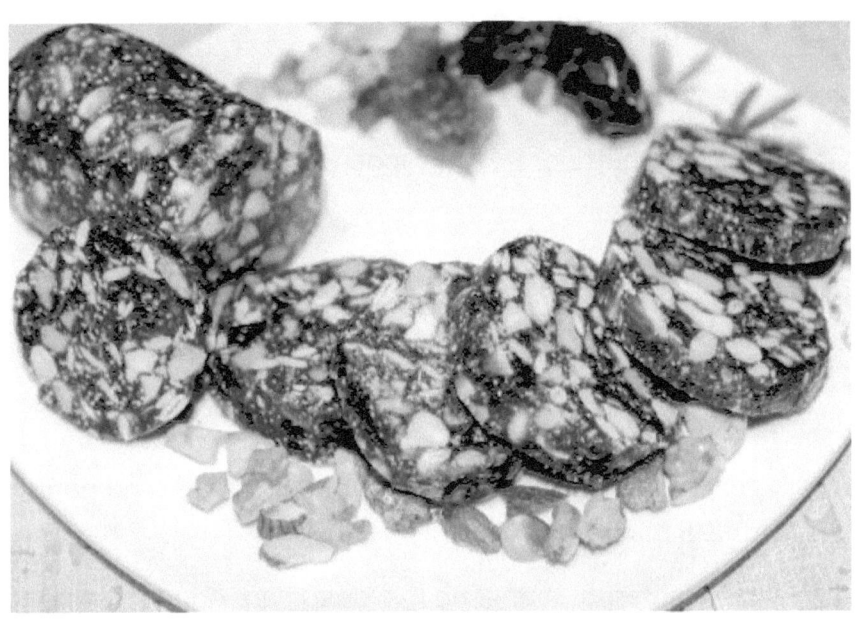

For 20 rolls

Ingredients:

Dates (deseeded): 1½ cup

Dried figs: ½ cup

Almonds: ¼ cup

Cashews: ¼ cup

Walnuts: ¼ cup

Pistachio: ¼ cup

White sesame: 1 tablespoon

Melon seeds: 1 tablespoon

Pumpkin seeds: 1 tablespoon

Poppy seeds: 1 teaspoon

Ghee (Clarified butter): 1½ tablespoons

Method:

1. Chop almonds, cashews, walnuts, and pistachio finely.

2. Grind dates and fig without using any water.

3. Dry roast sesame, melon seeds, pumpkin seeds, and poppy seeds for 3-5 mins.

4. Warm ½ tablespoon of ghee in a deep pan. Add all the nuts and roast in low flame until they slightly turn brown and release an aromatic smell.

5. Remove the nuts from heat. Add 1 tablespoon of ghee to the same pan.

6. Add dates and fig mixture. Mix well. Cover with a lid and let it soften for about 2 minutes.

7. Remove the lid and cook for about 5-7 min. Add nuts and seeds to it. Mix well and bind the mixture together by pressing it with a spatula.

8. Turn off the flame. Let it cool for 2 min. Take out the mixture on a plate. Grease your palm with ghee so that the mix doesn't stick to your palm. Now give the mixture a cylinder shape. Wrap it in with a cling film. Refrigerate the roll for 1 hour.

9. Take out the roll from the fridge. Remove the cling film. Grease a knife and cut the roll into small pieces.

10. Store in a clean and dry place for up to 2 weeks.

READ THE COMPLETE SERIES

Read the complete Eat So What! Mini Editions Series:

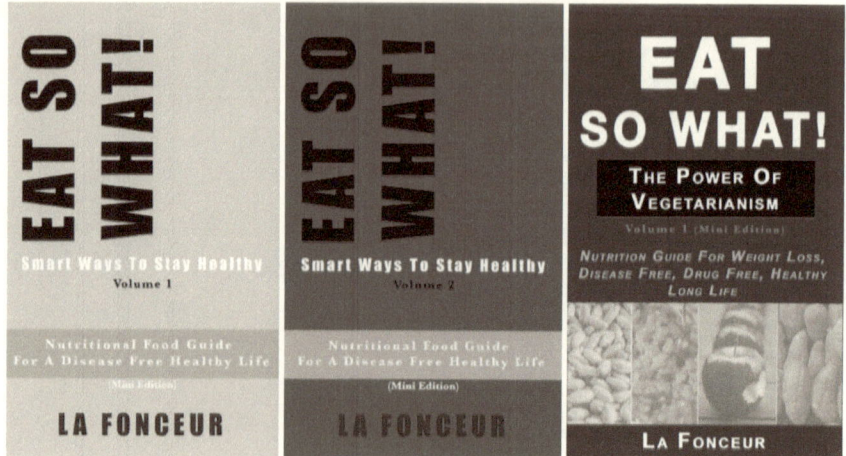

Book 1   Book 2   Book 3

ABOUT THE AUTHOR

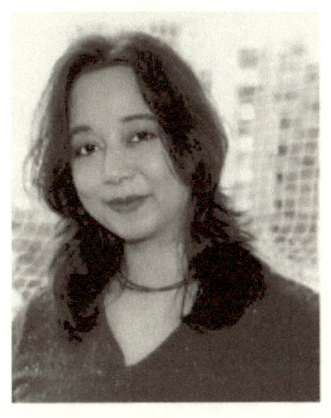

La Fonceur is the author of the book series *Eat So What!*, *Secret of Healthy Hair*, and *Eat to Prevent and Control Disease*. She is a health blogger and a dance artist. She has a master's degree in Pharmacy. She specialized in Pharmaceutical Technology and worked as a research scientist in the research and development department. She has published an article titled "Techniques for Producing Biotechnology-Derived Products of Pharmaceutical Use" in the Pharmtechmedica Journal. She is also a registered pharmacist. Being a research scientist, she has worked closely with drugs. Based on her experience, she believes that one can prevent most diseases with nutritious vegetarian foods and a healthy lifestyle.

NOTE FROM LA FONCEUR

Dear Reader,

Thank you for reading *Eat So What! The Power of Vegetarianism Volume 2*. I hope you have found this book helpful.

If you liked the book, please leave a short review onlinetelling why you enjoyed reading it. This will help other health-conscious readers find this book. Your help in spreading awareness is gratefully received.

Join my mailing list at www.eatsowhat.com/esw-newsletter to receive updates on my new release.

_____

Also, read how foods that work with the same mechanism as medicines can naturally prevent and control disease in *Eat to Prevent and Control Disease*.

If you are looking for a permanent solution to your hair problems, read *Secret of Healthy Hair*.

All of my books are available in eBook, paperback, and hardcover editions. Happy reading!

Regards

La Fonceur

ALL BOOKS BY LA FONCEUR

Full-length books:

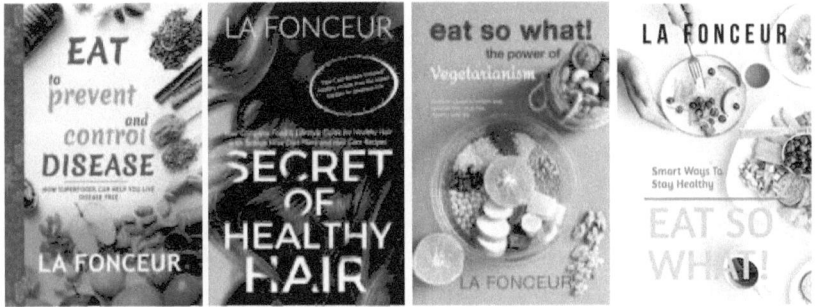

Mini extract editions:

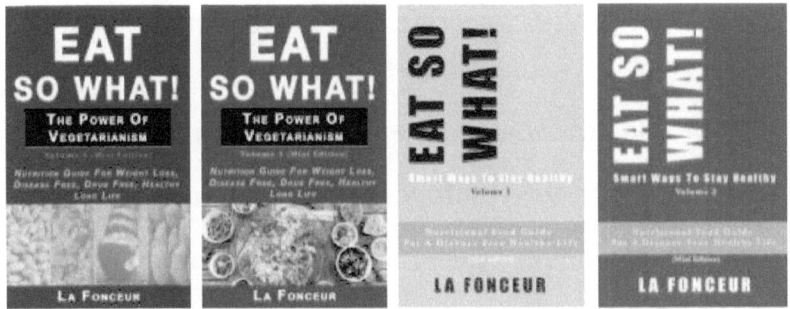

Hindi editions:

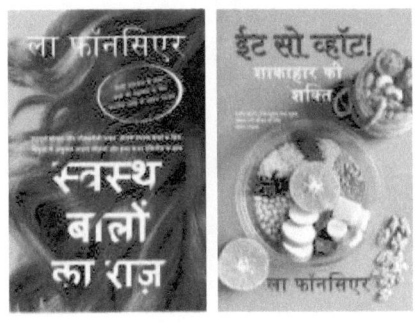

CONNECT WITH LA FONCEUR

Instagram: **@la_fonceur** | **@eatsowhat**

Facebook: **LaFonceur** | **eatsowhat**

Twitter: **@la_fonceur**

Amazon Author Page:

www.amazon.com/La-Fonceur/e/B07PM8SBSG/

Bookbub: **www.bookbub.com/authors/la-fonceur**

Sign up to the websites to get exclusive offers on La Fonceur eBooks:

Health Blog: **www.eatsowhat.com**

Website: **www.lafonceur.com/sign-up**

www.ingramcontent.com/pod-product-compliance
Lightning Source LLC
Chambersburg PA
CBHW020356290526
45785CB00005B/2319